Fruit Infused

101

Natural Vitamin

Water Recipes

By

Jamie Watson

Table of Contents

CHAPTER 3: TROPICAL FRUIT INFUSED WATER 22

CHAPTER 4: GO LOCO OVER COCO VITAMIN WATER40

CHAPTER 5: BERRY DELICIOUS WATER   48

CHAPTER 6: CITRUS BURST   60

INTRODUCTION

I want to thank you and congratulate you for downloading the book, *"Fruit Infused Water: 101 Natural Vitamin Water Recipes"*.

This book contains different vitamin water recipes without additives. You will get to drink nothing but natural vitamin water that is good for your health. It is also economical and you can share it with your entire household. It is quick and easy to prepare. You can store your homemade vitamin water in the fridge for three days, but with these delicious recipes you will surely want to immediately gulp it down to the last drop.

You can serve vitamin water to guests and refill your pitcher up to four to five times, depending on the remaining flavor of the ingredients in your pitcher. It is recommended to refill your pitcher when it is already half empty to get a flavor intensity that's almost the same as that of the previous batch. Expect the flavor to go milder as you refill your pitcher.

It is also important to wash your ingredients well and peel your fruit to avoid bitter-tasting water. If you want more flavorful vitamin water, then you can include the peelings (put the peelings in the water after peeling your fruit) but remember to take them out after two to three hours of infusion. If you don't peel your fruit and just soak it in the water for two to three hours and then remove it, then expect your vitamin water to taste bland. The fruit slices will continue to give additional flavor in your water if you let them stay as you refill. That's why it is wise to peel your fruit prior to soaking.

You can try different recipes of vitamin water in one day and share it with family or friends. Prepare your vitamin water the way it should be done and expect flavorful encounters in the days to come.

Thanks again for downloading this book, I hope you enjoy it!

CHAPTER 1: REFRESHING MINT WATER

RASPBERRY MINT AND ORANGE WATER

Ingredients:

1½ cups raspberries, lightly mashed
1 orange, peeled and sliced
½ cup mint leaves, lightly crushed
2 quarts water
2 cups crushed ice

How to prepare:

Put the ingredients in the pitcher, except ice and water. Muddle the ingredients for a bit; add your crushed ice followed by water. Put the pitcher inside the refrigerator and infuse for at least three hours. Treat yourself to a refreshing drink.

CHERRY MINT WITH CUCUMBER

Ingredients:

Half cup of mint leaves, crushed
1 cup fresh cherries, pitted and halved
1 small cucumber, peeled and sliced
2 quarts water
1 cup crushed ice

How to prepare:

Put your cherries in the pitcher and lightly mash them. Put in the mint leaves and cucumber; muddle everything for a bit. Add the crushed ice and stir. Carefully pour the water as you continue stirring the ingredients. Infuse for four hours in your refrigerator. Serve.

COOL APPLE, STRAWBERRY, AND CUCUMBER BLEND

Ingredients:

Sprig of mint
2 apples, cored and quartered
1 medium-sized cucumber, peeled and sliced thinly
½ cup strawberries, sliced
2 quarts water
1 cup crushed ice

How to prepare:

Put your fruit slices in the pitcher. Mash the fruits lightly using a wooden spoon. Add crushed ice and stir. Pour the water into the pitcher and infuse for four hours in the refrigerator before serving.

LEMON-LIME AND MINT CUCUMBER WATER

Ingredients:

1 medium-sized cucumber, sliced thinly
2 lemons, peeled and sliced
2 limes, peeled and sliced
Sprig of mint, lightly crushed
2 quarts water
1 cup crushed ice

How to prepare:

Put all the ingredients in the pitcher, except water. Muddle for a bit before adding the water. Infuse for three hours in the refrigerator before serving. You can add lemon juice for a more intense flavor.

REFRESHING MANGO AND ORANGE

Ingredients:

1 orange, peeled and sliced (you can save ¼ orange to squeeze into the water)
1 ripe mango, peeled and sliced
2 sprigs of mint, lightly crushed
2 quarts water
1 cup crushed ice

How to prepare:

Arrange your fruit slices and herb in the pitcher. Add crushed ice and stir using a muddler. Squeeze some orange juice. Add water in the pitcher and infuse for an hour at room temperature and for another three hours in the refrigerator. Serve and enjoy your drink.

SIZZLING LIME AND CUCUMBER WATER

Ingredients:

2 cucumbers, peeled and sliced thinly
1 lime, peeled and quartered
4 chilies with seeds intact, chopped (add more chilies if you want it spicier)
2 quarts water
1 cup crushed ice

How to prepare:

If you want your water to be less spicy, then you can

remove the seeds of the chili. The chili seeds are the ones responsible for giving the heat. Put all your ingredients in the pitcher except crushed ice and water. Mix the ingredients well using a wooden spoon. Add ice and water. Infuse for an hour at room temperature and for two hours in the refrigerator. Strain the seeds as you pour your vitamin water in a glass.

PEACH AND PLUM IN SPARKLING WATER

Ingredients:

1 to 2 peaches, sliced
1 plum, sliced
1 long sprig of mint, lightly crushed
1 quart sparkling water
2 cups crushed ice

How to prepare:

Put the herb, fruits, and crushed ice in the pitcher. Mix everything in your pitcher. Pour the water and put the pitcher insider the refrigerator. Infuse for three to four hours (or overnight) before serving. You can garnish your drink with peach slices if you want. Enjoy your vitamin water.

CHERRY MINT IN SPARKLING CUCUMBER WATER

Ingredients:

1 medium-sized cucumber, peeled and sliced thinly
1 cup cherries, pitted and halved
Sprig of mint, lightly crushed
1 quart sparkling water
2 cups crushed ice

How to prepare:

Arrange your ingredients in the pitcher and muddle using a wooden spoon. Add crushed ice and sparkling water; stir everything together. Infuse at room temperature for an hour before putting the pitcher in the refrigerator to infuse for another three hours. Serve in a fancy glass and enjoy.

ORANGE MINT AND PINEAPPLE

Ingredients:

1 orange, peeled and sliced
1 cup pineapple (you can use canned pineapple), diced
1 sprig of lavender, lightly crushed
1 sprig of mint, lightly crushed
2 quarts water
1 cup crushed ice

How to prepare:

Put your fruits and herbs in the pitcher. Add the crushed ice and muddle for a bit. Add water and put the pitcher in the refrigerator. Let it infuse for three hours before serving.

PEACH MANGO AND MINT WATER

Ingredients:
15 slices of peach (frozen)
1 ripe mango, sliced
1 long sprig of mint
2 quarts water
1 cup ice

How to prepare:

Put the fruits in the pitcher and muddle for a bit using a wooden spoon. Add the sprig of mint and crushed ice, and mix the ingredients well. Pour in the water and stir. Put your pitcher in the fridge and let it stay there for at least four hours before you pour yourself a drink.

MINT CANTALOUPE AND LIME WITH A TWIST

Ingredients:

3 cups cantaloupe, peeled and diced

2 limes (get the juice of one and slice the other one)
2 tablespoons fresh mint leaves, lightly crushed
1 pinch salt
1 to 2 tablespoons honey
2 quarts water in a separate pitcher
2 cups crushed ice

How to prepare:

Add the honey in a pitcher with water, and stir well. You can also add in the salt. In another pitcher, combine the rest of the ingredients and muddle for a bit to release the flavor. Pour in the water, together with salt and honey; stir well. Infuse for an hour at room temperature and another two hours in the refrigerator. Serve when ready.

CITRUS FRUIT AND PEAR WITH HOT GREEN PEPPER

Ingredients:

1 tangerine, peeled and sliced
1 Meyer lemon, peeled and sliced
1 bunch cilantro
1 pear, peeled and sliced
1 hot green pepper (add more if you want it spicier), sliced
2 quarts water
2 cups crushed ice

How to prepare:

Put the ingredients in the pitcher, except the last two on the list. Get your wooden spoon and muddle the ingredients in the pitcher for a bit. Add in the crushed ice followed by water. Infuse at room temperature for an hour and for another three hours in the refrigerator. Serve and enjoy your drink.

MINTY APPLE WITH PLUM AND BLUEBERRIES

Ingredients:

1 cup blueberries, lightly smashed
1 plum, sliced
1 apple, cored, and sliced
1 sprig of mint, lightly crushed
2 quarts water
2 cups crushed ice

How to prepare:

Put the fruits and mint in the pitcher. Slightly mash the ingredients using your wooden spoon. Add ice, and then water. Put the pitcher in the refrigerator and infuse for three hours.

THIRST-QUENCHING CUCUMBER AND WATERMELON MINT WATER

Ingredients:

1 medium-sized cucumber, peeled and sliced
2 cups watermelon, diced
1 sprig of mint, lightly crushed
2 quarts water
2 cups crushed ice

How to prepare:

Put the watermelon and cucumber in the pitcher and smash a little. Add in the mint and mix everything well. Add in the crushed ice and water; stir well. Infuse for an hour or two then serve.

CHAPTER 2: GINGER ALL THE WAY

INVIGORATING GINGER AND PEAR COMBO

Ingredients:

1 piece of 1-inch-long ginger, peeled and sliced thinly
2 pears, sliced thinly
2 quarts water
2 cups crushed ice

How to prepare:

Put all the ingredients in the pitcher, except water. Stir the ingredients using a muddler. Pour in the water. Let it infuse for one hour at room temperature, and for four hours more in the refrigerator. Strain and pour the clear water into your glass.

LEMON GINGER WITH LAVENDER

Ingredients:

2 medium-sized lemons
1 sprig lavender
1 piece of 2-inch-long ginger, peeled and grated

2 quarts water

1 cup crushed ice

How to prepare:

Get one of the lemons and cut it in half. Squeeze the lemon half, get the juice, and put the juice in the pitcher. Slice the remaining lemon and lemon half. Put all the ingredients in the pitcher, except water. Mix your ingredients and add water. Infuse at room temperature for an hour and then put the pitcher in the refrigerator and infuse for another three hours. Serve and enjoy your drink.

CUCUMBER AND LEMON IN GINGER WATER

Ingredients:

1 piece ginger (about 2 inches long), peeled and grated

2 lemons, peeled and sliced

1 small cucumber, peeled and sliced

½ cup mint leaves, slightly crushed

2 quarts water in a separate container

1 cup crushed ice

How to prepare:

Put the grated ginger in the container with water and stir for a bit; set aside. Put the remaining ingredients in the pitcher and stir using a muddler or wooden spoon. Pour in the ginger water and stir once more. Put the pitcher in the refrigerator and infuse for at least four hours.

BANANA-ORANGE COMBO IN GINGER WATER

Ingredients:

2 oranges, peeled and sliced
1 ripe banana, peeled and sliced
1 piece of 1-inch-long ginger, peeled and grated
2 quarts water in a container
2 cups crushed ice

How to prepare:

Put the grated ginger in 2 quarts water. Put all the other ingredients in the pitcher and stir. Pour the water with ginger over the ingredients in the pitcher. Put the pitcher in the refrigerator and infuse for four to five hours. Serve and enjoy.

ZESTY GINGER ORANGE WATER

Ingredients:

2 medium-sized mandarin oranges, peeled and sliced
1 piece 1-inch-long ginger, peeled and sliced

2 quarts water

1 cup crushed ice

How to prepare:

Put the orange and ginger in your pitcher. Get your wooden spoon and muddle a little. Add the crushed ice followed by water. Enjoy a refreshing drink.

RASPBERRY, LEMON, AND CUCUMBER GINGER WATER

Ingredients:

1 medium-sized cucumber, peeled and sliced thinly

1 lemon, peeled and sliced

1 cup raspberries, lightly smashed

1 piece 2-inch-long ginger, peeled and sliced

7 pieces mint leaves, torn by hand

2 quarts water

1 cup crushed ice

How to prepare:

Put all the ingredients in the pitcher except the last two on the list. Use a muddler to release the flavors of the ingredients in the pitcher. Add crushed ice, stir, and pour water in the pitcher. Put the pitcher in the refrigerator and let the flavor infuse for four hours. You can pour yourself a drink after the infusion.

ORANGE-CANTALOUPE IN GINGER WATER

Ingredients:

1 orange, peeled and sliced into wedges or rings
1 cup cantaloupe, peeled and diced
1 piece 2-inch-long ginger, peeled and grated
2 quarts water in a container
1 cup crushed ice

How to prepare:

Mix the grated ginger in the water; set aside. Put the diced cantaloupe in the pitcher and mash lightly, and add the orange slices followed by the crushed ice. Mix the ingredients well and pour in the water with ginger. Put the pitcher in the refrigerator and infuse for two to four hours. Serve and enjoy your drink.

BLOOD ORANGE AND BASIL IN GINGER WATER

Ingredients:

2 blood oranges, peeled and sliced
1 piece 2-inch-long ginger, peeled and grated
2 quarts water in a separate pitcher
2 cups crushed ice

How to prepare:

Put the grated ginger in the pitcher with 2 quarts water; set aside. Get another pitcher and put all the other ingredients in. Muddle the ingredients for a bit using your muddler or wooden spoon. Pour in the water and infuse in the refrigerator for three hours.

GINGER CINNAMON APPLE DELIGHT

Ingredients:

1 stick cinnamon
1 apple, cored and sliced
1 piece 2-inch-long ginger, peeled and grated
1 quart sparkling water
2 cups crushed ice

How to prepare:

Put cinnamon, apple, ginger, and crushed ice in the pitcher and muddle for a bit. Add in the sparkling water and stir to blend the flavors. Put the pitcher in the fridge and infuse for two to four hours. Enjoy your sparkling drink.

GINGER PINEAPPLE MANGO MIX

Ingredients:

2 cups pineapple, peeled and coarsely chopped

1 ripe mango, peeled and diced
1 piece 2-inch-long ginger, peeled and grated
2 quarts water in a separate pitcher
1 cup crushed ice

How to prepare:

Add the grated ginger in the 2 quarts water; set aside. In another pitcher, put in all the remaining ingredients and mix well. Pour in the water with ginger and infuse for four hours in the fridge. Serve and enjoy.

BERRY PASSIONATE GINGER WATER

Ingredients:

1 cup berries (your choice)
1 passion fruit, extract the seeds
1 piece 2-inch-long ginger, peeled and grated
2 quarts water
2 cups crushed ice

How to prepare:

Put the seeds of the passion fruit in a sieve and put the sieve in a bowl. Mash the seeds using a fork and get the juice. Combine the crushed ice, ginger, and berries in the pitcher. Mash the berries a little and pour the water in the pitcher; stir. Add the passion fruit juice and the seeds. Mix everything well and put the pitcher in the fridge to infuse the flavor. Allow it to stay in the fridge for four hours. Serve and enjoy your refreshing drink.

PINEAPPLE PASSION

Ingredients:

2 passion fruit (cut in half and extract the seeds)
1 piece 2-inch-long ginger, peeled and grated
2 cups pineapple, peeled and chopped
2 quarts water in a separate pitcher
1 cup crushed ice

How to prepare:

Put the grated ginger in the pitcher of the 2 quarts water; set aside. Get another pitcher and put all the other ingredients in. Muddle the ingredients for a bit using your muddler or wooden spoon. Pour in the water and infuse in the refrigerator for three hours.

TROPICAL MANGO CLEMENTINE WITH GINGER

Ingredients:

1 cup ripe mango, peeled and coarsely chopped
1 Clementine, peeled and sliced
1 piece 1-inch-long ginger, peeled and sliced

2 quarts water

3 cups crushed ice

How to prepare:

Put the mango, ginger, crushed ice, and Clementine in the pitcher. Get your wooden spoon and mix your ingredients well. Add the water in the pitcher and infuse for 1 hour at room temperature and for 2 hours more in the in the refrigerator.

CHAPTER 3: TROPICAL FRUIT INFUSED WATER

MELON LYCHEE IN CUCUMBER WATER

Ingredients:

1 small cucumber, peeled and diced
1 cup cantaloupe, peeled and diced
2 cups honeydew, peeled and sliced
1 cup watermelon, peeled and diced
1 cup lychee, slightly mashed
2 quarts water
1 to 2 cups crushed ice

How to prepare:

Put the cucumber, melons, and lychee in the pitcher. Muddle for a bit and add crushed ice; mix well. Pour the water in the pitcher and infuse for four hours in the refrigerator.

BLUEBERRY HONEYDEW WATER

Ingredients:

2 cups blueberries, slightly mashed
1 cup honeydew, peeled and coarsely chopped
2 quarts water
1 cup crushed ice

How to prepare:

Put the fruits in the pitcher and mix well. Add crushed ice and water. Stir the ingredients well and put the pitcher in the refrigerator. Infuse for at least two hours before pouring yourself a drink.

PINE GUAVA AND CUCUMBER

Ingredients:

2 ripe guavas, peeled and sliced
1 cup pineapple, peeled and coarsely chopped
1 medium-sized cucumber, peeled and sliced thinly
1 sprig of lavender
2 quarts water
1 cup crushed ice

How to prepare:

Put all your ingredients in the pitcher, except water. Mix everything in the pitcher before pouring in the water. Infuse in the refrigerator for three hours. Serve and share.

Cool Blue Lychee with Pineapple

Ingredients:

1 cup ripe pineapple, peeled and coarsely chopped
½ cup blueberries, cut in half
1 cup lychee, slightly mashed
2 quarts water
1 cup crushed ice

How to prepare:

Arrange the lychee, berries, pineapple, and crushed ice in the pitcher. Muddle the ingredients using a wooden spoon to release the flavor. Add the water and stir. Put the pitcher in the refrigerator and infuse for at least two hours.

MINTY STRAWBERRY WATERMELON AND CUCUMBER

Ingredients:

1½ cup watermelon, peeled and cubed
1 cup strawberries, sliced
1 medium-sized cucumber, peeled and sliced
1 sprig of mint, slightly crushed
2 quarts water
1 cup crushed ice

How to prepare:

Arrange all ingredients in the pitcher, except water. Muddle gently using your wooden spoon. Pour the water into the pitcher and infuse for at least three hours in the refrigerator. Share and enjoy.

COOL MELON DEW

Ingredients:

2 cups honeydew, peeled and cubed
1 cup cantaloupe, peeled and coarsely chopped
1 cup watermelon, peeled and cubed

½ lemon, peeled and sliced
1 sprig of mint
2 quarts water
1 cup crushed ice

How to prepare:

Arrange all your fruits and herb in the pitcher. Muddle a little using a wooden spoon and add crushed ice and water. Mix everything well. Put the pitcher in the refrigerator and infuse for two hours. Serve, share, and enjoy.

CRANBERRY AND APPLE WITH CINNAMON

Ingredients:

1 apple, cored and sliced
1 cup cranberries, lightly mashed
1 stick cinnamon
2 quarts water
2 cups crushed ice

How to prepare:

Line all ingredients in your pitcher, except water. Slightly mash your apples using a wooden spoon. Add water and mix everything well. Put the pitcher in the fridge and infuse for four hours. Give yourself a treat afterwards.

SPARKLING GRAPEFRUIT AND WATERMELON WITH ROSEMARY

Ingredients:

2 cups watermelon, peeled and coarsely chopped
2 sprigs of rosemary, slightly crushed
1 grapefruit, peeled and sliced
1 quart sparkling water
2 cups crushed ice

How to prepare:

Put your fruits and herb in the pitcher and combine well. Add crushed ice and mix. Pour the sparkling water in the pitcher and stir. Infuse for an hour at room temperature; put the pitcher in the refrigerator and infuse for another two hours. Serve and enjoy.

TROPICAL PAPAYA AND LEMO-LIME

Ingredients:

1 cup ripe papaya, peeled and cubed
1 lime, peeled and sliced
1 lemon, peeled and cut in wedges
2 quarts water
1 cup crushed ice

How to prepare:

Put everything in your pitcher and stir. Let the pitcher sit at room temperature for an hour and put it in the refrigerator for three hours. After three hours, pour some vitamin water into your favorite glass. Enjoy your drink.

GRAPE, HONEYDEW, AND CANTALOUPE COOLER

Ingredients:

2 cups seedless grapes, halved
2 cups cantaloupe, peeled and cubed
2 cups honey dew, peeled and coarsely chopped
1 quart sparkling water
1 cup crushed ice

How to prepare:

Mix your ingredients in a pitcher, except the sparkling water. Mash the cantaloupe and honeydew for a bit to release their flavors. Pour sparkling water over the ingredients in the pitcher and infuse for four hours in the refrigerator. Enjoy a refreshing drink.

KIWI WATERMELON WITH BASIL

Ingredients:

2 cups watermelon, peeled and coarsely chopped
1 kiwi, peeled and sliced
6 basil leaves, coarsely shredded by hand
2 quarts water
1 cup crushed ice

How to prepare:

Combine all of the ingredients in the pitcher, except water. Mix well and add water. Put the pitcher in the fridge and infuse for three hours. Serve and enjoy your drink with friends.

CHERRY APPLE WITH CILANTRO

Ingredients:

2 apples, cored and sliced
1 bunch cilantro, coarsely chopped
½ cup cherries, pitted and halved
2 quarts water
2 cups crushed ice

How to prepare:

Put your fruits and herb in the pitcher and muddle or a bit. Add the ice and mix well. Add water in the pitcher and stir. Let it sit at room temperature for thirty minutes and infuse in the refrigerator for three hours. Enjoy your day with your flavorful and refreshing drink.

PINEAPPLE ORANGE WITH PASSION FRUIT

Ingredients:

1 passion fruit, scoop out the seeds
1 cup fresh pineapple, coarsely chopped
1 orange, peeled and sliced
1 quart sparkling water
2 cups ice

How to prepare:

Put the passion fruit seeds, pineapple, and orange into your pitcher. Mix them well. Add in ice and water. Stir to combine the flavors well. Put it in the refrigerator and infuse for at least four hours.

PEACH MANGO VANILLA

Ingredients:

2 peaches, peeled and sliced
1 cup ripe mango, peeled and diced
1 vanilla bean, cut in half
2 quarts water
1 cup crushed ice

How to prepare:

Put all of the ingredients in the pitcher except the last two on the list. Gently mash your peaches using your muddler, add crushed ice, and mix everything well. Add water and infuse for four hours in the refrigerator. Enjoy a refreshing drink.

APPLE AND PERSIMMON WITH ROSEMARY

Ingredients:

2 apples, cored and sliced
1 persimmon, peeled and sliced
1 sprig of rosemary, slightly crushed
2 quarts water
1 cup crushed ice

How to prepare:

Arrange your fruits in your pitcher and mash lightly. While mixing the ingredients, add in rosemary and crushed ice followed by water. Infuse for four hours in the fridge. Serve among friends and enjoy your afternoon.

TROPICAL MANGO AND PERSIMMON COOLER

Ingredients:

1 persimmon, peeled and sliced
1 ripe mango, peeled and sliced
2 quarts water
1 cup crushed ice

How to prepare:

Put your fruits and crushed ice in the pitcher; mix well. Pour the water over the ingredients and put the pitcher in the refrigerator. Infuse for three hours or more. Pour some vitamin water in a glass after three hours and enjoy your drink.

MANGO AND ORANGE WITH BASIL

Ingredients:

1 large ripe mango, peeled and sliced
1 orange, peeled and sliced
A handful of basil, torn
2 quarts water
1 cup crushed ice

How to prepare:

Arrange the mango and orange slices in the pitcher. Add basil and mix well. Add crushed ice followed by water. Leave it on the table at room temperature for an hour. Put the pitcher in the refrigerator and infuse for two hours more. Serve to your guests or family.

ATERMELON AND RASPBERRY ROSEMARY

Ingredients:

2 cups watermelon, peeled and coarsely chopped
1 cup raspberries, lightly mashed
2 long sprigs of rosemary, slightly crushed
2 quarts water
1 cup crushed ice

How to prepare:

Arrange the watermelon, rosemary, and raspberries in the pitcher. Add crushed ice on top. Add enough water to cover the ingredients. Let it sit for thirty minutes. Add the remaining water and infuse for three hours in the fridge. Get a nice glass and pour yourself a drink.

APPLE, GRAPEFRUIT, PINEAPPLE, AND PAPAYA MEDLEY

Ingredients:
1 small apple, cored and sliced
1 grapefruit, peeled and sliced
1 cup ripe papaya, peeled and diced
1 cup pineapple, peeled and diced

2 quarts water
2 cups crushed ice

How to prepare:

Put the ingredients in the pitcher, except water. Mix them well. Add water and stir. Let it sit at room temperature for about an hour and put the pitcher in the refrigerator. For more flavorful vitamin water, infuse for four hours in the fridge. After such time, you can get your favorite glass and pour yourself a refreshing drink.

APPLE AND CITRUS MIX

Ingredients:

1 apple, cored and sliced
1 Clementine, peeled and sliced
1 cup pineapples, peeled and cubed
1 pear, cored and sliced
2 quarts water
2 cups crushed ice

How to prepare:

Put your fruits in the pitcher and muddle for a bit. Add ice and water; mix well. Infuse for two to four hours in the fridge. Serve and enjoy your drink.

PINEAPPLE CRANBERRY COOLER

Ingredients:

1 cup fresh pineapple, peeled and cubed
¾ cup cranberries, cut in half
1 stick cinnamon
2 quarts water
1 cup ice

How to prepare:

Put the ingredients in your pitcher, except ice and water. Muddle your ingredients using your wooden spoon. Add ice and water in the pitcher. Put the pitcher in the fridge and infuse for at least two hours before serving.

PINEAPPLE MANGO MINT COOLER

Ingredients:

1 cup fresh pineapple, peeled and sliced
1 ripe mango, peeled and sliced
1 sprig of mint
2 quarts water
1 cup ice

How to prepare:

Put the fruits in your pitcher together with crushed ice and mint. Muddle for a bit. Add water and stir. Place the pitcher in the refrigerator and infuse for at least three hours. Serve and enjoy.

PEAR, APPLE, AND PERSIMMON

Ingredients:

2 pears, cored and sliced
1 apple, cored and sliced
1 persimmon, peeled and sliced
1 lemon, peeled and sliced
2 cinnamon sticks

2 quarts water

1 cup crushed ice

How to make it:

Put the fruits and crushed ice in your pitcher and muddle for a bit. Add water and cinnamon sticks in the pitcher. Put the pitcher in the fridge and infuse for four hours. Serve and enjoy with the whole family.

BANANA NECTARINE WITH BASIL

Ingredients:

1 ripe banana, peeled and sliced

1 nectarine, peeled and sliced

1 handful of basil, torn in two

2 quarts water

1 cup ice

How to prepare:

Put all the ingredients in the pitcher, except water; mix well. Add water and infuse for an hour at room temperature. Put the pitcher in refrigerator and infuse for another three hours.

APPLE AND PEAR AND EVERYTHING NICE

Ingredients:

1 apple, cored and sliced
1 plum, sliced
1 cup blueberries, cut in half
1 pear, cored and sliced
1 lemon, get the juice
1 sprig of mint
2 quarts water
1 cup ice

How to prepare:

Put everything in the pitcher, except ice and water. Muddle for a bit using a wooden spoon. Add ice and water, and infuse for four hours in the fridge. Serve with lemon slices if you want.

PINEAPPLE LYCHEE MINT COOLER

Ingredients:

1 cup fresh pineapple, peeled and sliced
1 cup lychee, peeled and slightly mashed
1 sprig of mint, lightly crushed
2 quarts water
1 cup ice

How to prepare:

Put everything in the pitcher. Muddle for a bit and place the pitcher in the fridge. Infuse for at least two hours. Serve and enjoy.

CHAPTER 4: GO LOCO OVER COCO VITAMIN WATER

BERRIES AND APRICOT IN COCONUT WATER

Ingredients:

1 cup raspberries, cut some in half

1 cup blackberries, cut some in half
1 apricot, peeled and sliced
2 cups crushed ice
1 quart water
1 liter coconut water

How to prepare:

Put the berries and apricot in the pitcher. Muddle for a bit and pour the coconut water over your ingredients. Add the crushed ice and water. You can use 2 liters of coconut water and don't add plain water anymore. Infuse for at least two hours in the fridge.

COCO MELON, PERSIMMON, AND ORANGE MEDLEY

Ingredients:

1 orange, peeled and sliced
1 persimmon, peeled and sliced
1 cup melon, peeled and diced
1 sprig of mint, slightly crushed
1 cup coconut water
2 quarts water
1 cup crushed ice

How to prepare:

Put the fruits, herb, and coconut water in the pitcher. Mix them well. Add in the crushed ice and water. Infuse for two hours in the refrigerator. Enjoy your healthy and refreshing water.

LEMON AND BERRIES COCO COOLER

Ingredients:

1 medium-sized lemon, peeled and sliced
1 cup raspberries, slightly mashed
1 cup cranberries, slightly mashed
1 liter coconut water
1 quart plain water
1 cup crushed ice

How to prepare:

Combine the berries, lemon, and coconut water in the pitcher. Muddle for a bit, and then add crushed ice. Stir and add plain water. Put the pitcher in the refrigerator and infuse for two hours.

LIME AND CHERRY IN COCONUT WATER

Ingredients:

1 lime, peeled and sliced thinly
1 cup cherries, pitted and halved
600 ml coconut water
2 cups crushed ice

How to prepare:

Combine the lime slices and cherries in the pitcher, and add coconut water; stir. Add crushed ice and infuse at room temperature for an hour. Put the pitcher in the refrigerator and infuse for one hour. Enjoy your fruit-infused coco water.

HONEYDEW AND BLUEBERRY IN COCONUT WATER

Ingredients:

½ cup blueberries, cut in half
1 cup honeydew, peeled and diced

600ml coconut water
1 cup crushed ice

How to prepare:

Arrange your berries and honeydew in the pitcher. Mash them lightly. Add the crushed ice and coco water. Put the pitcher in the fridge and infuse for two hours.

RASPBERRY AND LEMON IN COCO WATER

Ingredients:

½ cup raspberries, sliced
1 lemon, peeled and sliced
600ml coconut water
1 cup crushed ice

How to prepare:

Put all the ingredients in the pitcher and muddle for a bit. Let it sit at room temperature for thirty minutes and another two hours in the fridge. Enjoy your drink in your favorite tall glass.

CHEERY CHERRY, APPLE, AND LIME

Ingredients:

1 cup pitted cherries
1 lime, peeled and sliced
1 apple, cored and sliced
600ml coconut water
1 quart water
1 cup crushed ice

How to prepare:

Line the fruits in your pitcher. Get your wooden spoon and smash them gently. Add the coconut water and stir. Add the crushed ice and plain water. Put the pitcher in the fridge and infuse for three hours. Treat yourself with a nice drink.

KIWI IN COCONUT WATER

Ingredients:

1 kiwi fruit, peeled and sliced
600ml coconut water
1 cup plain water
1 cup crushed ice

How to prepare:

Combine the coconut water and kiwi in the pitcher. Mix well and add crushed ice followed by plain water. Infuse for at least an hour. Serve and enjoy.

COCONUT WATER, CLEMENTINE AND BLUEBERRY

Ingredients:

½ cup blueberries, cut in half
1 Clementine, peeled and sliced
600ml coconut water
1 quart plain water
1 cup ice

How to prepare:

Mix Clementine, blueberries, and coconut water in the pitcher. Add crushed ice and plain water. Infuse for two hours in the fridge. Enjoy your refreshing coco water.

WATERMELON AND APRICOT WITH COCONUT WATER

Ingredients:

5 cups seedless watermelon, peeled and cubed
2 apricots, peeled and sliced
1 medium lime, get the juice
1 liter coconut water
1 quart plain water
1 cup ice

How to prepare:

Mix apricots, watermelon, lime juice, and coconut water in the pitcher. Add crushed ice followed by plain water; stir. Infuse for three hours in the refrigerator. Serve and enjoy a refreshing coco water treat.

CHAPTER 5: BERRY DELICIOUS WATER

BLUE CUCUMBER WITH BASIL

Ingredients:

1 cup blueberries, cut in half
1 cucumber, peeled and sliced
1 handful basil, torn
2 quarts water
1 cup ice

How to prepare:

Mix blueberries, cucumber, and basil in the pitcher. Add water and ice; stir. Infuse for four hours in the refrigerator. Enjoy your refreshing water.

BERRIES GALORE

Ingredients:

½ cup strawberries, quartered
½ cup blueberries, quartered
½ cup raspberries, quartered
½ cup blackberries, quartered

2 quarts water
1 cup crushed ice

How to prepare:

Line the berries in your pitcher and mash them lightly using your wooden spoon. Add ice (crushed) and water into the pitcher. Infuse for two hours or more but not more than twelve hours.

BLUE CRANBERRY MERRY MIX

Ingredients:

1 cup blueberries, slightly mashed
½ cup cranberries, slightly mashed
1 medium-sized ripe banana, peeled and sliced
1 cup coconut water
2 quarts water
1 cup crushed ice

How to prepare:

Put the berries, banana, and coco water in the pitcher. Mix the ingredients well. Add crushed ice and water; stir. Put the pitcher in the fridge and infuse for four hours.

BERRY PINE BANANA BEETS WITH LEMON

Ingredients:

2 beets, peeled and sliced
1 lemon, peeled and cut in wedges
1 ripe banana, peeled and coarsely chopped
¼ cup strawberries, chopped
½ cup pineapple, peeled and diced
2 quarts water
1 cup crushed ice

How to prepare:

Put everything in the pitcher, except water. Mix the ingredients in the pitcher. Add water and stir for a bit before placing the pitcher in the refrigerator. Infuse for four hours.

HONEY BERRY ORANGE

Ingredients:

2 medium-sized oranges, peeled and sliced
½ cup honeydew, peeled and diced

1 cup cranberries, lightly mashed
2 quarts water
1 cup crushed ice

How to prepare:

Assemble the fruits at the bottom of the pitcher. Muddle for a bit before adding ice (crushed) and water. Infuse for two to three hours in the refrigerator. You can choose to add crushed rosemary if you want a bit of variety.

BLUE APPLE AND PLUM WITH COCO WATER

Ingredients:

2 apples, cored and sliced
2 plums, pitted and sliced
1 cup blueberries, sliced
1 cup coconut water
2 quarts water
1 cup crushed ice

How to prepare:

Arrange your fruits in the pitcher and add coconut water. Muddle for a bit using a wooden spoon. Add crushed ice and water, and infuse for three hours in the refrigerator. Serve and enjoy.

Peachy Mango with Blueberry

Ingredients:

½ cup blueberries, cut in half
2 peaches, pitted and sliced
1 ripe mango, peeled and sliced
2 quarts water
1 cup crushed ice

How to prepare:

Gather your fruits at the bottom of the pitcher. Lightly mash them together using a wooden spoon or muddler. Add crushed ice followed by water, and infuse for three hours in the refrigerator. Pour some vitamin water in a glass and enjoy.

Apple and Cranberry with Peach

Ingredients:

3 apples, cored and sliced
1 cup cranberries, lightly mashed
1 peach, peeled and sliced
2 quarts water
1 cup crushed ice

How to prepare:

Put all ingredients into your pitcher, except water. Slightly mash them using your muddler. Add water and put the pitcher in the fridge to infuse for four hours. Serve and enjoy.

REFRESHING BERRIES AND MINT

Ingredients:

1 cup cranberries, sliced
1 cup blueberries, sliced
½ raspberries, lightly mashed
1 sprig of mint
2 quarts water
1 cup crushed ice

How to prepare:

Arrange the fruits and mint in your pitcher, and muddle a little. Add crushed ice and water. Put the pitcher in the refrigerator to infuse for two hours. Serve and enjoy.

BLACKBERRY MAGIC WITH MINT LIME

Ingredients:

1 cup blackberries, cut in half
1 sprig of mint, lightly crushed
1 lime, peeled and sliced
2 quarts water
1 cup crushed ice

How to prepare:

Arrange your berries and herb in the pitcher. Muddle for a bit. Add crushed ice, water, and lime slices. Infuse for four hours in the fridge. Enjoy your drink.

BLUE GRAPES AND CUCUMBER

Ingredients:

1 cucumber, peeled and sliced
½ cup grapes, cut in half

1 cup blueberries, cut in half

2 quarts water

2 cups crushed ice

How to prepare:

Put the ingredients in the pitcher, except water. Mix the ingredients well. Add water and infuse for four hours in the fridge.

BLOOD ORANGE AND CUCUMBER COOLER WITH RASPBERRY

Ingredients:

1 medium-sized cucumber, peeled and sliced

½ cup raspberries, lightly mashed

1 blood orange, peeled and sliced

2 quarts water

1 cup ice

How to prepare:

Arrange your fruits in the pitcher. Muddle for a bit with a wooden spoon. Add ice and water in the pitcher. Infuse for at least two hours in the fridge.

ROSEMARY ORANGE WITH CRANBERRY

Ingredients:

1 orange, peeled and sliced
1 cup cranberries, lightly mashed
1 sprig of rosemary, lightly crushed
2 quarts water
1 cup ice

How to prepare:

Line your fruits and herb in the pitcher; mix them well. Add water and crushed ice over your ingredients. Put the pitcher in the fridge and infuse for four hours.

RASPBERRY LEMON IN COCONUT WATER

Ingredients:

1 lemon, peeled and sliced
½ cup raspberries, cut in half
2 cups coconut water
1 quart water
1 cup ice

How to prepare:

Combine all the ingredients in the pitcher. Let it sit at room temperature for an hour and for another two hours in the fridge. Drink and enjoy.

BLACKBERRY, RASPBERRY, AND LIME WITH MINT WATER

Ingredients:

1 cup blackberries, sliced
½ cup raspberries, lightly mashed
1 sprig of mint, lightly crushed
1 lime, peeled and sliced
2 quarts water
1 cup crushed ice

How to prepare:

Combine all the ingredients in the pitcher, except water. Muddle for a bit before you add water. Infuse for four hours in the refrigerator. Serve and enjoy.

STRAWBERRY, RASPBERRY, AND ORANGE IN SPARKLING WATER

Ingredients:

1 cup strawberries, sliced
½ cup raspberries, lightly mashed
1 orange, peeled and sliced
1 quart sparkling water
1 cup crushed ice

How to prepare:

Add the fruits and crushed ice in the pitcher and muddle. Add sparkling water and infuse in the refrigerator for four hours.

RASPBERRY AND BLUEBERRY WITH GINGER AND COCO WATER

Ingredients:

1 cup raspberries, lightly mashed
1 cup blueberries, cut in half
1 piece 1-inch-long ginger, peeled and sliced
2 cups coconut water
1 quart plain water
1 cup ice

How to prepare:

Mix the ingredients in the pitcher, except plain

water. Add water and stir. Put the pitcher in the refrigerator and infuse for at least two hours. Serve and enjoy.

CHAPTER 6: CITRUS BURST

AMAZING DETOX WATER

Ingredients:

1 medium-sized cucumber, peeled and sliced
½ cup cranberries, lightly mashed
2 lemons, peeled and sliced
1 bunch parsley, coarsely chopped
1 bunch cilantro, coarsely chopped
2 quarts water
2 cups crushed ice

How to prepare:

Put the fruits and herbs in the pitcher and muddle for a bit. Add crushed ice and stir. Add water and infuse for an hour at room temperature. Put the pitcher in the fridge and infuse for three hours more. Feel clean and fresh after a drink.

GOOSEBERRY AND LEMON MINT WATER

Ingredients:

½ cup gooseberries, seeds removed and fleshed

scooped out
1 lemon, peeled and halved
2 sprigs of mint, lightly crushed
½ teaspoon salt
2 quarts water
1 cup crushed ice

How to prepare:

Get half of the lemon and squeeze the juice into the pitcher. Thinly slice the other half and add into the pitcher. Add the gooseberries, salt, and mint. Add crushed ice and water in the pitcher and stir. Infuse for four hours in the fridge.

STRAWBERRY, GRAPEFRUIT, AND CLEMENTINE WITH SAGE

Ingredients:

2 cups grapefruit, peeled and sliced lightly mashed
1 Clementine, peeled and sliced
1 cup strawberries, sliced
3 teaspoon sage, ground
2 quarts water
1 cup crushed ice

How to prepare:

Put grapefruit in the pitcher and mash it lightly. Add strawberries, sage, and crushed ice; stir. Pour water over the ingredients and put the pitcher in the fridge. Infuse for at least two hours. Serve and enjoy a refreshing treat with friends.

BLUE POMEGRANATE IN SPARKLING WATER

Ingredients:

1 pomegranate
2 cups blueberries, cut in half and lightly mashed
1 piece 1-inch-long ginger, peeled and sliced
2 quarts water
1 cup crushed ice

How to prepare:

Cut pomegranate into quarters and submerge the slices in a bowl of water. Strain the seeds and add them in the pitcher. Add the other ingredients, except water. Muddle for a bit and add water. Infuse for at least two hours in the refrigerator.

ORANGE AND GRAPEFRUIT SURPRISE

Ingredients:

1 orange, peeled and sliced
2 cups grapefruit, peeled and sliced
1 small ripe banana, peeled and sliced thinly
1 cup cantaloupe, peeled and diced
2 quarts water
1 cup crushed ice

How to make it:

Put the citrus fruits in the pitcher and mash lightly. Add banana, cantaloupe, and crushed ice; muddle for a bit. Pour your water over the ingredients and infuse for at least three hours in the refrigerator before serving.

GRAPEFRUIT FLAVOR EXPLOSION

Ingredients:

2 cups grapefruit, peeled and sliced into small pieces
1½ cup ripe banana, peeled and sliced
1 orange, peeled and sliced
1 cup strawberries, sliced
2 quarts water
1 cup crushed ice

How to make it:

Combine all your ingredients, except water. Muddle for a bit. Add water over the ingredients and infuse for two hours in the fridge. Serve and enjoy.

APPLE AND PERSIMMON WITH CELERY AND LIME

Ingredients:

3 apples, cored and sliced
2 medium-sized carrots, peeled and sliced
1 persimmon, peeled and sliced
2 limes (get the juice of one lime, and peel and slice the other one)
1 stalk of celery, sliced (remove the root part)
2 quarts water in a container
1 cup crushed ice

How to prepare:

Put the lime juice in the water and add the slices of apple and persimmon. Combine the remaining ingredients together in the pitcher. Add in the water with apple and persimmon slices. Muddle a little and infuse for three hours in the fridge.

LEMON GINGER APPLE WITH COCONUT WATER

Ingredients:

2 medium-sized beets, peeled and sliced
1 piece 1-inch-long ginger, peeled and grated
1 lemon, peeled and sliced
1 apple, cored and cubed
2 cups coconut water
2 quarts water
1 cup crushed ice

How to prepare:

Gather your ingredients in the pitcher, except water. Mix well and add water. Let it sit at room temperature for an hour. Infuse for two hours more in the refrigerator.

PEAR TANGERINE WITH CILANTRO AND MEYER LEMON

Ingredients:

1 pear, cored and sliced
1 tangerine, peeled and sliced
1 Meyer lemon, peeled and sliced

1 bunch cilantro

2 quarts water

1 cup crushed ice

How to prepare:

Line the fruits and herb in your pitcher and gently muddle using a wooden spoon. Add water and crushed ice to the mixture. Infuse for about four hours in the fridge. Your drink is ready.

PINEAPPLE AND ORANGE BURST WITH CUCUMBER

Ingredients:

1 Clementine, peeled and sliced

1 cup pineapple, peeled and diced

1 blood orange, peeled and sliced

1 tangerine, peeled and sliced

1 cucumber, peeled and sliced

2 quarts water

1 cup crushed ice

How to prepare:

Combine all the ingredients in the pitcher, except water. Mix them well and add water. Stir a little and put the pitcher in the refrigerator to infuse for four hours. Serve and enjoy.

LEMON AND LIME WITH CILANTRO

Ingredients:

2 lemons, peeled and sliced
1 lime, peeled and sliced
1 bunch cilantro
2 quarts water
1 cup crushed ice

How to prepare:

Put your fruits and herb in the pitcher. Mash gently using a wooden spoon. Add water and let it sit in the refrigerator for four hours. You can add some honey if you want.

KIWI WITH CANTALOUPE AND LAVENDER

Ingredients:

2 ripe kiwis, peeled and sliced

¼ cup lavender leaves, lightly crushed
1 cup cantaloupe, peeled and diced
2 quarts water
1 cup crushed ice

How to prepare:

Combine kiwi, cantaloupe, and lavender in the pitcher. Mix the ingredients well. Add crushed ice and water. Put the pitcher in the refrigerator to infuse for four hours. Serve and enjoy.

LEMON AND PLUM WITH WATERMELON

Ingredients:

1 lemon, peeled and sliced
4 plums, pitted and sliced
1 cup watermelon, peeled and cubed
2 quarts water
1 cup crushed ice

How to prepare:

Put the fruits in your pitcher and muddle with a wooden spoon. Add water and crushed ice. Let it sit in the refrigerator for four hours to infuse.

CITRUS EXPLOSION

Ingredients:

1 blood orange, peeled and sliced
1 lemon, peeled and sliced
1 cup grapefruit, peeled and cut into small pieces
1 lime, peeled and sliced
1 cup cantaloupe, peeled and coarsely chopped
2 quarts water
1 cup crushed ice

How to prepare:

Combine all the ingredients in the pitcher, except water. Get a wooden spoon and muddle for a bit. Add water and infuse for two hours in the refrigerator.

ORANGE ROSEMARY WITH LIME COCONUT WATER

Ingredients:

1 orange, peeled and sliced
1 lime, peeled and sliced
1 sprig of rosemary, slightly crushed

2 cups coconut water

2 quarts water

1 cup ice

How to prepare:

Arrange the fruits in the pitcher and muddle for a bit. Add water and infuse for four hours in the refrigerator. Enjoy your drink with family and friends.

CHAPTER 7: FLOWER IN THE WATER

Before trying different flowers to include in your water, take note that you need to use the flowers that are known to be safe to eat. If you are uncertain, then you need to check first before jumping in.

Choose organic flowers or those that were not treated with chemicals or pesticides. Do not use flowers from a flower shop that might have been treated with chemicals. The same goes for flowers that you can see at the park or by the roadside.

It is recommended to consume or use only the petals, and cut off the stamens and pistils. To keep them fresh, you can put them on moist paper towels and store them in your fridge. Make sure to put them in an airtight container.

EXOTIC ORANGE HIBISCUS FLAVORED WATER

Ingredients:

3 Mandarin oranges, peeled and sliced
1 tablespoon hibiscus flowers
2 quarts water
1 cup ice

How to prepare:

Mix all the ingredients in a pitcher. Put the pitcher in the refrigerator and infuse for four to five hours. Strain the ingredients after four or five hours. Enjoy your flowery drink.

Take note that hibiscus (and other flowers) must not be over-infused in the water because it can leave an overwhelming taste.

BLACKBERRY ROSE WITH VANILLA WATER

Ingredients:

¾ cup blackberries, lightly mashed
¼ cup pink rose petals, dried
½ of vanilla bean, cut lengthwise
2 quarts water
1 cup ice

How to prepare:

Mix everything in a pitcher. Put the pitcher in the fridge and infuse for at least three hours. Strain the ingredients before serving your exotic water.

RASPBERRY VANILLA ROSE WATER

Ingredients:

½ cup raspberries, lightly mashed
½ of vanilla bean, cut lengthwise
1 handful organic rose petals, fresh (remove the white base because it is bitter, use only the petals)
2 quarts water
1 cup ice

How to prepare:

Mix everything in a pitcher. Put the pitcher in the fridge and infuse for at least three hours. Strain the ingredients before serving your exotic water.

BLUEBERRIES WITH LAVENDER FLOWER POWER

Ingredients:

1 cup blueberries, lightly mashed
1 handful lavender
2 quarts water
1 cup ice

How to prepare:

Mix everything in a pitcher. Leave at room temperature for an hour. Put in the refrigerator to infuse for two hours. Serve and enjoy.

SWEET CARNATION WITH BLUEBERRIES

Ingredients:

1 cup blueberries, lightly mashed
1 handful carnation
½ peach, peeled and sliced
2 quarts water
1 cup ice

How to prepare:

Put the peach slices in the pitcher and lightly mash. Add the remaining ingredients in the pitcher; stir. Put the pitcher in the refrigerator to infuse for at least two hours. Serve and share among friends.

CHRYSANTHEMUM AND BLUEBERRIES

Ingredients:

1 cup blueberries, lightly mashed
1 handful chrysanthemum
2 quarts water
1 cup ice

How to prepare:

Chrysanthemum is somewhat bitter; expect the flavor to range from peppery to pungent, depending on the variety of mum you will use. Combine everything in a pitcher and infuse for four hours in the refrigerator. Serve and enjoy.

CONCLUSION

Thank you again for downloading this book!

I hope this book was able to give you the flavor that you have been looking for in your vitamin water.

The next step is to try the different recipes and share them with the people you hold dear.

Finally, if you enjoyed this book, please take the time to share your thoughts and post a review. It'd be greatly appreciated!

Thank you and good luck!

DID YOU ENJOY THIS BOOK?

I want to thank you for purchasing and reading this book. I really hope you got a lot out of it.

Can I ask a quick favor though?

If you enjoyed this book I would really appreciate it if you could leave me a positive review on Amazon.

I love getting feedback from my customers and reviews on Amazon really do make a difference. I read all my reviews and would really appreciate your thoughts.

Thanks so much.

Jamie Watson

Printed in Great Britain
by Amazon